Sciatica No More

A Comprehensive Guide to Sciatica Causes, Symptoms, Treatments, and a Holistic System of Natural Remedies for Sciatica Pain Relief

Pamela H. Royal
Copyright© 2014 by Pamela H. Royal

Sciatica No More

Copyright© 2014 Pamela H. Royal

All Rights Reserved.
Warning: The unauthorized reproduction or distribution of this copyrighted work is illegal. No part of this book may be scanned, uploaded or distributed via internet or other means, electronic or print without the author's permission. Criminal copyright infringement without monetary gain is investigated by the FBI and is punishable by up to 5 years in federal prison and a fine of $250,000. (http://www.fbi.gov/ipr/). Please purchase only authorized electronic or print editions and do not participate in or encourage the electronic piracy of copyrighted material.

Publisher: Enlightened Publishing

ISBN-13: 978-1499170009

ISBN-10: 1499170009

Disclaimer

The Publisher has strived to be as accurate and complete as possible in the creation of this book. While all attempts have been made to verify information provided in this publication, the Publisher assumes no responsibility for errors, omissions, or contrary interpretation of the subject matter herein. Any perceived slights of specific persons, peoples, or organizations are unintentional.

This book is not intended for use as a source of legal, business, accounting or financial advice. All readers are advised to seek services of competent professionals in the legal, business, accounting, and finance fields.

The information in this book is not intended or implied to be a substitute for professional medical advice, diagnosis or treatment. All content contained in this book is for general information purposes only. Always consult your healthcare provider before carrying on any health program.

Table of Contents

Introduction: My Story 5

Chapter 1: What is Sciatica? 13

    Sciatica Nerve Pain 14

    Descriptions of Sciatica Pain 16

    Psychosomatic Sciatica 18

Chapter 2: Sciatica Diagnostic Processes 21

    Physical Examination 22

    Spine X-ray 23

    Electromyography 23

    Myelography 24

    MRI 24

Chapter 3: Common Causes of Sciatica 27

Chapter 4: Non-Surgical Treatment Options 35

    Exercises and Therapy 35

    Car Seat Cushions 37

    Sensible Footwear 37

Sciatica Shoes and Insoles 39

Sciatica Back Braces 39

Popular Exercises 41

Acupuncture 45

Ice and Heat 46

Knowledge Therapy 48

Inversion Table 49

Decompression Therapy 51

Epidural Steroid Injections (ESIs) 52

TENS for Sciatica 53

Chapter 5: Natural Remedies 55

Hypnosis 55

Yoga 56

Reiki 57

Biofeedback 57

Massage Therapy 58

Naturopathy, Homeopathy, Herbal Medicine 58

Chapter 6: Surgical Treatment Options 61

Back Surgery 61

Failed Back Surgery Syndrome 63

Chapter 7: Medications for Sciatica Pain 65

Over-the-counter Pain Relief Medications 66

Prescription Drugs 66

Natural Pain Relief for Sciatica 67

Chapter 8: Working with Sciatica Pain 69

Creating Ideal Posture for the Office......... 69

Long Periods of Standing............................. 71

Chapter 9: Travelling with Sciatica Pain 73

Before You Travel.. 74

Waiting for Transportation.......................... 76

During a Flight 77

Travelling by Car 78

Chapter 10: Sleeping with Sciatica Pain 81

The Right Mattress.. 81

The Right Position... 83

Chapter 11: Myths and Facts about Sciatica . 85

Summary: Learn to Say Sayonara Sciatica 87

Introduction: My Story

I woke up one morning and could not get out of bed – literally. Every time I attempted to raise myself to a sitting position, pain shot through my lower back and into my left hip and buttock.

Eventually, after much thought and reasoning, I finally rolled onto my stomach, slid off the bed onto my hands and knees, and crawled into the bathroom. Once there, I gingerly hoisted myself onto the side of the tub and into a sitting position, which would enable me to somehow slide onto the commode. Finally, I had arrived.

Now that I was in a sitting position, I began to ponder my next challenge, which would be getting back to the bedroom and into bed. With my feet flat on the floor and sitting on a hard surface, I discovered that I could stand if I placed one hand on the small of my back and the other hand on the side of the vanity. (I really think the hand on the back was just to help me feel as though I had support.)

Having stood, I could slide my feet across the floor and inch my way back to the bed. I remember standing there, looking at the bed and feeling like it was a huge, formidable obstacle.

Eventually, I decided to stand with my side to the bed and ease down on my right buttock, keeping my back as straight as possible. Since the pain was mostly on the left side, that proved to be a good decision.

Once there, I rolled onto my right side and gradually inch-wormed myself back into bed.

Horrors! What was I to do? I needed to get to the medicine cabinet for pain relief meds, which I didn't want to take on an empty stomach, which meant that I also needed to eat, at least, a light breakfast.

I needed to pull out the heating pad, and I needed some type of topical pain relief applied to my back. Last but not least, I need to call my job and step them through everything someone else would need to do that day. But all I wanted to do was lie very still and pray that the pain would end as quickly as it had come – but it didn't.

The previous day, I had shoveled dirt into two holes, which were each about 2 feet square. I had been feeling wonderful. My weight was good and I was getting regular exercise. Nothing strenuous, but lots of walking.

Years prior, I had experienced back pain resulting from a fall. I knew that I should avoid heavy lifting and that snow shoveling was a big no-no. The real problem, however, for me, was that when I felt well, I tended to forget the need to be cautious and mindful of my back condition. When I felt well, I envisioned myself as some kind of super person.

Well, after two or three days of bed rest and no improvement, I went to see my doctor. He examined me and said that I was suffering from classic sciatica symptoms. He then ordered an MRI of my back. The MRI revealed a moderate sized herniated disk (also called a compressed disk). My doctor then sent me to a pain management specialist.

During this time, I continued to be in pain. I had begun to loathe my car because sitting was excruciating. There were days when I went to work, closed my office door, and laid on the floor just to get a little relief.

I was on prescribed pain medications and had begun taking an over-the-counter medication that actually helped with the pain. Being hypertensive, I had regularly scheduled routine blood work. On one such occasion, the blood analysis revealed high liver enzymes, indicating that the pain medication was having an adverse effect on my liver. My doctor said I had to discontinue taking the medication.

The specialist recommended spinal injections and physical therapy, but he cautioned me that he would only do 4 injections during the course of a year. The first injection, which I found extremely painful, helped a little at first, but the pain came back. I started physical therapy three times a week, but the pace was too fast and too strenuous and always caused a setback.

After about eight weeks of constant pain and no improvement, I began to analyze my condition. I realized that in an effort to avoid pain, I had shorted my stride when I walked. I also realized that I was doing as few physical activities as possible (other than that excruciating therapy).

Meanwhile, my doctor recommended a second spinal injection and told me that if I didn't get better, he would send me to a surgeon. I was determined that surgery would be my absolute last resort and that I had to come up with a plan. Mind you, however, that I was not offered any other solutions.

I discontinued physical therapy, but did the exercises faithfully in the morning and evening. I did them at my pace and comfort level. Following each exercise period, I applied ice to my back for 15 to 20 minutes. I also started walking around the block once every day. It didn't matter how long it took, as long as I walked.

I focused on lengthening my stride because I knew that by now, my hamstrings had to be extremely tight, which was placing tension on my back. It hurt to take bigger strides, but eventually, it got easier.

I envisioned my tendons lengthening and relieving the lower back tension. I envisioned the mechanics of my back -- one bulging disk and another pancake flat -- and I imagined them shifting into proper alignment. I imagined my muscles becoming stronger and supporting my back.

Finally, after 12 weeks of discomfort, the pain was subsiding. The pain management specialist was amazed and maybe even slightly unbelieving. He firmly reiterated that if the pain came back, I would definitely need to see a surgeon, to which I firmly responded, "Dr. Lee, the pain will not be coming back."

That was six years ago. I have not needed to see a healthcare professional for sciatica back pain since then. I continue to care for my back with stretching, walking and sometimes back strengthening exercises. Oh, and every now and then, I also treat my back to spinal decompression at the chiropractor's office.

Why I Wrote This Book

I believe our bodies were designed to heal. I believe that each of us has a personal responsibility to become armed with knowledge about our conditions and that we need to listen to our bodies. Medical professionals are wonderful, but you are the only person who knows how you feel.

The single most important thing I learned through my ordeal with sciatica is that there is no way any doctor can tell every patient everything he or she needs to know and, unfortunately, most patients don't know what questions to ask.

I am hoping that this book will help people learn about their conditions, learn of the many treatment options, learn to live within the limitations of their bodies and learn to live free from sciatica pain.

12

Chapter 1: What is Sciatica?

The word *sciatica* actually means that the sciatic nerve is experiencing pressure by one of the structures in the spine. Sciatica refers to symptoms, not a disease. These symptoms are characterized by pain and sometimes, numbness in areas of the body where the sciatic nerve is located. Other types of sciatic discomfort include weakness and tingling.

The sciatic nerve is the largest nerve in the body. It begins in the lower back and extends through the buttock, thigh and calf, finally ending at the foot. The location of the pain varies depending on what portion of the sciatic nerve is affected by injury, inflammation or abnormal pressure.

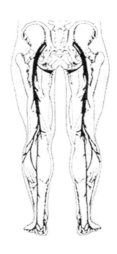

Sciatica Nerve Pain

Because of the many possible causes of sciatica, there are varying degrees and durations of sciatica pain. Sometimes recovery can occur within a few weeks or it may take several months or even longer. Depending on the cause of the pain, it may only be mild and irritating; or it may be absolutely unbearable.

The different types of sciatica nerve pain usually involve one or more of the following:

- Ongoing pain which occurs in one buttock or leg (usually not in both buttocks)

- More pronounced pain when sitting

- A burning or tingling sensation in the leg

- Feeling of numbness or weakness of the leg or foot

- Sharp pain caused by standing or walking

Have you ever heard anyone say, "I woke up this morning and couldn't get out of bed."? Sciatic pain can be so severe that the only relief is to remain absolutely still.

Of course, people in pain tend to avoid activities or movement that will cause more pain. The problem with this is that immobility may eventually cause other problems that will only make it more difficult to recover from sciatica.

It is of vital importance to visit your healthcare professional in order to get a correct diagnosis. Once a diagnosis has been made and the cause of the pain determined, your physician will be able to recommend treatment options.

Descriptions of Sciatica Pain

Listed below are descriptions of common types of sciatica pain:

Unilateral Sciatica

Unilateral sciatica is when pain occurs only on one side of the body. This type of sciatica pain is often predictable and is commonly caused by a structural problem. Diagnosis is easier when pain is consistently experienced the same way and in the same area of the body.

Bilateral Sciatica

With Bilateral sciatica, pain is felt on both sides of the body, although, not necessarily at the same time. Bilateral sciatic pay may occur alternatively from one leg to the other or one leg may experience greater pain. Typically, the pain is similar to that which is felt with unilateral sciatica.

Sciatica Foot Drop

When a person has difficulty or is unable to lift the front portion of the foot, this is called foot drop. Being able to lift the foot is necessary for walking and other daily functions. In sciatica patients, this condition is often caused by herniated discs or bone spurs in the spine, otherwise known as spinal osteophytes.

Sciatica Stiffness

Muscle stiffness is another manner in which sciatica pain is presented. With sciatica stiffness, the muscles feel cramped and tight. Muscle stiffness often accompanies other forms of sciatica pain and is sometimes caused when the muscle experiences oxygen deprivation.

Sciatica Constipation

Constipation is one of a very few non-spinal conditions that can cause sciatica. The sciatic nerve can become irritated even when using the bathroom. Since compression of the sciatic nerve causes sciatica pain, it is not unusual for constipation to be at the root of the problem.

Burning Sciatica

When sciatica pain is accompanied by the feeling or sensation of heat in the back, buttocks, legs or feet, it is referred to as burning sciatica. Sometimes this is a constant feeling of spasms of heat that course through the lower limbs. It can be actual heat or just the sensation of heat and may be an indication of muscle or nerve involvement.

Pregnancy Sciatica

Sciatica pain, especially during the third trimester of pregnancy, is not uncommon. As the uterus expands and the fetus grows, the additional weight and pressure can cause sciatic nerve inflammation. During the third trimester, as the baby shifts into the birth position, it may press directly against the nerve, resulting in sciatic pain.

Psychosomatic Sciatica

Because of the mystery and often misunderstood nature of psychosomatic illness, I felt that the topic of psychosomatic sciatica deserved its own little section.

Contrary to popular belief, the word 'psychosomatic' is not an indication that pain is imaginary. Actually, psychosomatic refers to true physical symptoms, but they are not caused by disease or illness.

These symptoms are the result of mind/body interactions. This is a defense mechanism of the subconscious mind designed to shield the conscious mind from having to resolve troublesome and/or highly sensitive thoughts, issues and feelings. The subconscious mind provides a way to keep the mind occupied on physical pain, while the actual source of the pain remains repressed and internalized.

The mind chooses pain because physical discomfort is all but impossible to ignore. People in severe pain are debilitated to the point where the pain is all-consuming. Typically, the level of physical pain is indicative of the emotional severity.

There are many ways in which the body and the mind interact. To name a few…

1. Fear can cause the heart to beat faster.

2. Sexual thoughts cause obvious body responses.

3. Nervousness can create butterflies in the stomach.

Although most people readily accept the existence of typical mind/body reactions, we often struggle with the ideal of psychosomatic pain and dismiss it as being unreal.

Unfortunately, a large portion of medical professionals is not trained in mind/body issues, which means that many times, psychosomatic pain is misdiagnosed. There are some healthcare professionals who are achieving positive results in the treatment of sciatica pain as psychosomatic illness. However, when psychosomatic pain is diagnosed as sciatica pain resulting from disease or injury, treatment will fail.

Medical treatment may provide temporary relief, but will not address the true source of the pain. For this reason, some patients' sciatica pain remains unresolved.

The misdiagnosis becomes a 'sciatica scapegoat'. You know the saying, "If it looks like a duck and quacks like a duck…" Since the symptoms so closely mirror sciatica pain caused by anatomical disease and injury, misdiagnosis is imminent unless the mind/body equation is considered.

Chapter 2: Sciatica Diagnostic Processes

There are several home remedies that may resolve mild sciatica pain. Some of these home remedies are rest, over-the-counter pain medications, ice and heat therapy and stretching exercises, or any combination. However, experiencing severe or persistent sciatica symptoms for a prolonged period of time is a strong indication that it is time to consult a physician for consultation and treatment.

After diagnosis, your health care professional may include some of these treatments along with his professional treatment plan. However, delay in seeing a physician getting a professional diagnosis could very well cause further complications.

A series of diagnostic tests are required to determine the cause of sciatica pain. The physician also needs to remove the possibility that the pain may only be lower back pain associated with muscle spasm or strain or something that is easily remedied. For example, pain in the lower back may also occur if one leg is shorter than the other. Heel lifts placed inside the shoe of the shorter leg may be an easy remedy for this condition and may prevent more serious outcomes.

Physical Examination

The patient's medical history is important because it may indicate if there is a disk herniation or other serious structural cause of the pain. The next step in diagnosing sciatica symptoms is a thorough physical examination with special attention being to the legs and spine.

Most likely, your physician will be checking reflexes and muscle strength and range of motion. The patient will be asked to perform several routine activities that may cause pain. The patient's response when performing these activities will aid in the diagnostic process.

Spine X-ray

An x-ray is a diagnostic tool that uses radiation to make pictures of the body's organs and bones. When a spine x-ray is taken, it provides detailed images of the spine and lumbar region.

During an x-ray, radiation passing through each type of body tissue causes the image to be displayed at varying shades, depending upon the type of tissue. For example, because of the high density of bones, most of the radiation is unable to pass through the bone, thus causing the bone to appear as a white image on the film. Less dense body tissues, like fat, muscle and tumors will appear as various darker shades.

Electromyography

In this test, electrical waves caused by skeletal muscle activity are recorded by passing an electric current through a nerve.

Myelography

In this test, the space between vertebrae is injected with contrast dye in order to enhance the outcome of an x-ray image.

MRI

Magnetic resonance imaging or MRI uses a magnetic field and radio pulses to make detailed pictures of virtually every internal body part. Radiation is not used to produce this type of image. Another key difference between an x-ray and an MRI is that the MRI is able to produce highly detailed pictures of body structures, making it easier for a physician to accurately diagnose the condition.

A spinal MRI shows the vertebrae, disks and spinal column. It also indicates the spaces in-between each vertebra, which is the area through which nerves pass.

What to expect in an MRI

A word to the wise… Even for those who do not suffer from claustrophobia, having an MRI in a 'closed' machine is very stressful. The patient is positioned at lower open end of a horizontal tube and very gradually inserted headfirst into the tube. When fully inserted, only the feet extending beyond the opening. The rest of the body is entirely enclosed.

There is very little space between the patient's face and the inside of the chamber. There may be a light and a fan somewhere in the upper portion of the machine. When the images are being taken, there is loud banging and clanging.

Sometimes your physician will prescribe a mild sedative for use prior to the procedure – sometimes not. Sometimes the technician will offer headphones and/or music – sometimes not. Having suffered through this procedure, my description is that it felt like being buried alive.

If I had to do this again, it would only be done in an 'open' MRI machine. The 'open' machine greatly reduces stress and the feeling of claustrophobia.

26

Chapter 3: Common Causes of Sciatica

Listed below are some of the more common causes of sciatica.

Obesity

Medical experts have concluded that excess body fat or obesity can lead to sciatica pain. People with excess body fat are vulnerable to sciatica because excess weight adds pressure to the spinal nerve. In addition, abdominal fat and muscle weakness do not adequately support the skeletal structure in the mid-section.

Obesity has long been recognized as a main contributor to sciatica pain in adults. Recent finds show that obesity is becoming a contributor to sciatica pain in young adults, as well.

Excessive sitting

Sitting increases pressure on the spine and excessive sitting may contribute to spinal degeneration. It is important to avoid sitting for long periods of time and to stand at regular intervals, which helps to avoid muscular stiffness and minor pain. While sitting, try to reposition often so that your weight distribution is varied.

Not only does excessive sitting cause sciatica pain, but in many cases, it continues to be a source of pain after diagnosis of sciatica pain has been made.

Crossing legs

People who typically cross the same leg all the time consistently place most of their weight on the same buttock. This means that excessive pressure is placed on the sciatic nerve on that side of the body. Alternating between both legs reduces placing consistent pressure on the same buttock. Ideally, it better to not cross the legs at all.

Poor Posture

Poor posture is a very prominent cause of sciatica pain. Improper posture when sitting or standing can also cause more damage. Instances of poor posture include:

- Jutting the head forward

- Rounding the shoulders

- Slouching

- Holding one shoulder higher than the other

- Failing to tuck in stomach and hold chest in upright position

- Uneven weight distribution on the legs

Idiopathic Sciatica

When the cause of sciatic pain is not known, it is referred to as idiopathic sciatica. Studies have shown that some patients with undiagnosed sciatica pain suffer from oxygen deprivation of the sciatic nerve and possibly the surrounding muscles.

Emotional Stress

Although not widely recognized, emotional stress has been known to contribute to disk herniation and disk degeneration. Studies have shown that an appreciable number of patients reported experiencing significant emotional stress right before their sciatica episodes began.

It is believed that emotional stress brings on a dominant nervous condition known as a nervous state of sympathy which affects the body. This state can lead to a decrease in blood flow to the muscles and organs. Muscles deprived of adequate blood flow become easily fatigued and tight.

It is further believed that this sympathetic state also causes an increase of a type of white blood cell that creates degenerative changes and inflammation in the disks and spine.

Injury

Back injury and even back surgery and/or resulting scar tissue can lead to many kinds of sciatica pain. More severe cases of sciatic pain may be caused by physical injury to the spine. Some of the most common injuries are listed below:

- **Herniated Disk**

    What is known as a disk provides cushion between the vertebrae. Sometimes referred to as a slipped disk, a herniated disk is a disk that has ruptured or has become thin. The disk contains a gel, which then pushes outward and protrudes from between the two vertebrae.

The damaged disk may cause a bulge, an extrusion or a protrusion. A herniated disk may cause leg pain may to be more severe than back pain. Sometimes a patient with a herniated disk will have no back pain at all.

However, when the disk has taken the form of extrusion, there is a high incidence of back pain because with extruding gel. In severe cases, the gel may actually become unattached from the disk. Fortunately, extrusion is not a common form of disk herniation.

- **Annular Ring Abnormalities**

The Annular Ring is the band of fibrous tissue surrounding and protecting the disk. This ring is highly susceptible to pain and sometimes the ring may develop tears. If a tear allows nerve fibers to grow into the disk, this will trigger pain.

- **Lumbar Degenerative Disk Disease or Spondylosis**

  Aging, as well as previous back injury and excessive wear, can cause osteoarthritis in spinal joints. In osteoarthritis, the cartilage between the joints is destroyed. In place of this cartilage, extra bone or bone spurs develop. Eventually, these changes can cause the spine to become less mobile and the spaces for spinal nerves may narrow. Also disks may become dry and begin to degenerate.

- **Spinal Stenosis**

  Spinal stenosis occurs when the openings within the spinal canal begin to narrow. This is the opening where spinal nerves leave the spinal column. Obviously, narrowing of the opening would naturally cause pain and inflammation. In addition, arthritis, inflammation and birth defects may cause spinal stenosis.

- **Scoliosis**

  Scoliosis is when the spine curves from side to side. Normal curvature of the spine is from back to front. Although, noticeable scoliosis never appears to be a mild condition, it usually does not raise neurological alarm and does not cause severe pain.

  Mild to moderate forms of scoliosis should be regularly monitored by a specialist. However, severe scoliosis may affect several areas of the body and cause widespread pain.

- **Spondylosis**

  When one lumbar vertebrae slips over another, this is called spondylosis

  In children, this condition is often caused by a birth defect. Arthritis or other degenerative disease is usually the cause of spondylosis in adults. Spondylosis typically responds better to rest than physical activity.

- **Arthritis and Inflammatory Conditions**

  Arthritis, which is stiffness and painful joint inflammation, may cause sciatica pain. This stiffness usually happens gradually over a period of time and may eventually result in fusion of the vertebrae.

- **Compression Fractures and Osteoporosis**

  Osteoporosis is when the bones experience a loss of calcium. Eventually, they bones become weak and fragile. Typically, there is little pain unless the osteoporosis causes the vertebrae to collapse. This collapse is known as a compression fracture. Walking and other routine activities may cause increased pain with this type of diagnosis.

Chapter 4: Non-Surgical Treatment Options

Most patients and physicians will consider conservative, non-surgical treatment options first. There are many options available depending upon what is causing the sciatica pain.

It should be noted that this information is not intended to replace physician care, but rather, to educate. Treatment should always be recommended, implemented and monitored by a qualified licensed healthcare professional.

Exercises and Therapy

At the onset of sciatica pain, most patients will want to rest for a day or two. At the onset, many doctors will prescribe short-term rest and anti-inflammatory medication. This is fine, but prolonged rest may actually make the pain worse. Without exercise, the spinal structures and back muscles begin to lose conditioning and become less able to provide back support. With this loss of muscle strength, strain and back injury are more likely to occur.

Physical exercise is often the first options considered because many patients benefit from an exercise regimen specifically designed to treat the cause of their specific sciatica pain.

Exercises and physical therapy help reduce sciatica pain by strengthening muscles, and relieving tension and pressure to the affected areas. Additionally, exercise also helps to prevent reoccurrences by providing conditioning. Another benefit of exercise is that it promotes blood circulation, which helps maintain proper nutrition and fluids to the discs.

Physical therapy may be prescribed by a physiatrist, chiropractor or certified athletic trainer. A spine specialist who treats sciatica and leg pain is also able to tailor and prescribe specific exercises. Any of these healthcare professionals is able to instruct the patient on how to properly execute these exercises.

Car Seat Cushions

One of the most common complaints from sciatica patients is pain while sitting or driving. Sciatica seat cushions are designed to help maintain proper posture. Since driving is a necessity for most adults, a seat cushion for the car may be a great way to address sciatica pain while preventing further strain on the back.

Seat cushions for the car are usually made of foam, sheepskin or an inflatable material, although some are filled with gel or water. They are also available in different shapes and sizes to provide custom fit. When purchasing a sciatica cushion, it is important that the patient select a cushion that is designed to relieve his or her particular type of sciatica pain.

Sensible Footwear

The fit and shoe style is very important for anyone suffering from sciatica pain and for those who are trying to maintain optimal back health. Shoes have been known to aggravate back pain.

Shoes play a major role in supporting the body because feet are the body's foundation. It is not unusual for the wrong type or fit of shoe to cause imbalance and problems with weight distribution. This can have a negative effect on posture and gait and may eventually cause pain in the back. This is why foot comfort, support and fit are so important when caring for the back.

High heels create the body to be misaligned and cause strain on the lower back. When the heel is elevated more than an inch and a half, it is impossible to walk in the correct position. High heels should only be worn as little as possible and should definitely not be worn for walking long distances.

Flip-flops do not provide enough support to the feet. This lack of support may cause strain to joints and tendons. A heel counter is a strip of leather that is placed at the back of the shoe. Shoes that do not have a heel counter are likely to cause foot pain if worn for long distance walking.

Not surprisingly, sneakers, even more so than shoes, provide the best heel support because they have a highly supportive heel counter. It is also important to consider shock absorption when purchasing footwear.

Sciatica Shoes and Insoles

There is much debate over the effectiveness of sciatica shoes. Sciatica insoles and shoes are custom designed to ease the burden of ongoing leg and back pain. They are available in a variety of styles and are reported to use of pain relieving mechanisms which are placed in the shoe sole. These shoes are, however, expensive and may only provide relief to a certain degree.

Sciatica Back Braces

There are many different opinions, pros and cons to using back braces for sciatica pain. Undoubtedly, back braces can definitely provide some pain relief and other benefits, as well. The problem, however, is that prolonged use of a back brace can reduce muscle tone and cause the back to become dependent upon external support.

Listed below are some short-term benefits of using a back brace.

- **Decrease of movement**

  Back braces reduce some spinal movement along with muscle flexing, although, they do not eliminate movement. For this reason, a brace may be best used at the onset of pain or injury to provide some pain relief, rather than for long-term use.

- **Proper posture**

  The purpose of a back brace is to provide support and improve posture. When wearing a back brace, the patient becomes more aware of posture and makes a conscious effort to maintain proper posture and body positions.

- **Pelvic and lower spine support**

  When a back brace is worn, the abdominal pressure increases and produces the effect of providing support around the entire waist.

Popular Exercises

In addition to pain relief, these exercises also stretch spine. Below are some of the exercises commonly used for stretching and strengthening of the spine.

Hamstring stretch

There are three thigh muscles and tendons to which the word hamstring refers. Most often the term is used to indicate the thigh muscles in the back of the leg or to tendons in the leg. When the hamstring muscle is tight, pelvic motion is limited and causes an increase in stress across the lower back.

Tight hamstrings can also interfere with correct posture. Stretching these muscles and tendons is vital to gradually lengthen the muscles and tendons and to promote agility and less stress in the lower back.

The importance of keeping the hamstrings elastic and supple cannot be stressed enough. There are several hamstring stretches from which to choose, two of which are provided below.

- Lying on your back, hold the ends of a towel in each hand and sling the towel around the bottom of the foot.

- While exhaling, use the towel to raise the leg as high as possible. If possible the leg should be raised to the extent that stretching is felt in the back of the leg.

- Hold the upraised position for two count

- Slowly lower the leg to the floor.

- Repeat the exercise with the other leg.

- Alternating from one leg to the other, repeat the exercise 8 to 10 times.

Single leg stretch

This is another exercise that will help with stretching the hamstrings

- Lying flat on the back, .grasp one knee and slowly pull it toward the chest.

- Keeping the other leg straight, breathe in while tightening the abdominal muscles and, slowly lift the straight leg as high as possible. This will cause a stretching sensation in the spine.

- Exhale and slowly return to starting position.

- Alternating from one leg to the other, repeat the exercise 8 to 10 times.

Pelvic rock

Pelvic exercises are great for strengthening the lower back muscles. The pelvic rock is one of many such exercises.

- Lying flat on the floor, bend the knees so that the thigh is perpendicular to the chest and place the hands on the knee-caps.

- Keeping the back pressed against the floor, inhale and slowly rock the knees up toward the chest. This will tilt the pelvis and rock the tailbone slightly off the floor.

- Hold the position for a 3 count.

- Exhale and slowly rock the knees back to the starting position.

- Repeat 10 times.

Half push up

- Lying face down on the floor, place each hand shoulder width, palms flat against the floor.

- Breathing in, slowly press against the floor, raising the chest and ribs. Try to keep the shoulders square.

- Maintain the position for a 3 count.

- Breathing out, slowly lower the ribs and chest to the floor.

Walking

Listed below are just two of the many ways in which walking may help alleviate low back pain and promote overall back health.

- Walking strengthens muscles in the lower half of the body. These muscles stabilize the spine and keep the body upright.

- Walking also promotes circulation, allowing the blood to carry bringing nutrition and oxygen to the muscles and remove toxins.

If, however, due to pain, walking is not well tolerated, there are lower impact exercises, such as water aerobics that may be more comfortable because water makes the body more buoyant. Listed below are some of the ways in which walking is beneficial to sciatica pain sufferers.

Stretching and walking, when done on a regular basis, help the body to obtain greater range of motion.

Acupuncture

The effectiveness of acupuncture for pain relief is widely debated. The Traditional Chinese Medicine (TCM) philosophy is based on the theory that pain and illness are caused when the flow of life energy, also known as chi, is blocked. Acupuncture asserts that when needles are inserted along the chi pathway, the flow of life energy is then restored to the correlating organ or function in the body. Acupuncture is based upon philosophy and is not scientifically proven.

Many who promote the use of acupuncture claim that it will either (a) provide symptomatic relief or (b) actually treat disease such as cancer, hypertension, etc.

In addition to these claims, there are a few who have altered from the original philosophy of acupuncture and claim that it can be used to bring pain relief by releasing endorphins through stimulating the nerve. Although this frame of thought is plausible, there is no proven evidence to support this theory.

Ice and Heat

Ice and heat are time tested standard treatments for pain, swelling, inflammation and consequently, healing. There is a cycle of pain, then muscle spasm that occurs repeatedly whenever there is injury involving tissue and muscle. Heat relaxes the nerves that send pain signals and cold causes the nerves to become numb.

Heat cools the muscle by increasing blood circulation. Conversely, the body's natural response to ice is to warm the area, by sending more blood to the area in which ice is applied. Increased circulation also provides nutrition and oxygen to the affected area and speeds removal of waste material from the cells.

In essence, both ice and heat increase blood flow and promote healing. By properly applying heat and ice consistently over a period of time, the cycle of spasm and pain is broken, after which, healing begins.

Listed below are basic guidelines for using ice and heat to treat sciatica back pain. If the pain covers a wide area, such as the buttock, thigh, and calf, the ice and heat should be applied to the source of the pain.

- Ice should always be applied at the first indication of injury. Regardless whether the injury is caused by a chronic condition or trauma, it should be placed on the affected area immediately. This is very important. The sooner ice is applied, the better the chance of fast recovery. At least for the first day or two, apply ice every 20 minutes.

- After the initial period, stretching and other appropriate exercises can be started. Heat or ice should be applied before and after exercise. Either may be used. Many people use heat before exercise because it helps to relax the muscle. They follow up with ice after exercising. Whether heat or ice, the outcome is the same. Red blood cells are bombarding the area to aid the healing process.

Knowledge Therapy

Knowledge therapy has been used in cases where conventional treatments for sciatica back pain have failed. Knowledge therapy teaches the patient what is causing the pain and then how to end it.

This portion works hand-in-hand with the section of this report that refers to psychosomatic sciatica

We all recognize the effect the mind has on the body and vice versa. They are always in contact with one another. Even medications prescribed for the body respond to the contact between body and mind.

It has also been established that the body's unresponsiveness to treatment may well be the result of misdiagnosed psychosomatic pain. In this case, it is imperative that healthcare professionals consider the link between mental distress and pain.

Inversion Table

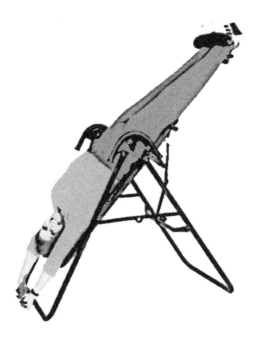

Any type of therapy that involves inverting the body to assist decompression of spinal bones is called inversion therapy. An inversion table positions the body on a slant with the head lower than the feet. Some exercises also incorporate this position and may provide other health benefits, as well.

Consultation with a healthcare professional is always recommended before participating in any kind of inversion therapy. Though inversion therapy is a healthy treatment option for people with disk compression, **those who or pregnant or who suffer from hypertension, glaucoma or heart disease are placed at increased risk of complication by using inversion.**

Because inversion therapy causes increased blood flow to the upper extremities, it also increases pressure in the eyeball. There are, however, safe, modified versions of this type of therapy that can be used at the advice of a healthcare professional.

Additionally, yoga positions that invert the body, such as headstands and shoulder stands, can inflict stress on the bones in the neck and should be only done in moderation.

Inversion therapy stretches the vertebrae which increases space between the bones of the spine. This reduces pressure and, thus, sciatica pain.

There are other benefits to inversion therapy, as well. When the head is positioned lower than the feet, it gives the heart muscle a chance to rest because of gravity is working with blood circulation. The heart does not have to work as hard because it is not pumping blood up the body. In addition, there is a nerve in the throat, that when nourished with blood, causes relaxation and stress reduction.

It is a common belief that inversion therapy is more effective for short-term relief than long term. Some healthcare professionals recommend inversion therapy for temporary pain relief, in addition to other forms of treatment.

Decompression Therapy

Spinal decompression is widely used in the treatment of sciatica pain. During spinal decompression, the spine is adjusted several times, causing the spine to relax. Spinal decompression causes a vacuum effect by using negative pressure to suck disk contents back inside the disk. This vacuum also promotes blood flow to the area, providing nutrition and oxygen, hence healing.

As with any treatment, decompression should only be implemented after diagnosis of the root cause of the pain.

Stiffness is a possible side effect of spinal decompression. **Also someone who is preg-**

nant cannot have decompression therapy because it causes pressure to the abdomen. Patients with osteoporosis and fusions of the vertebrae should avoid spinal decompression as it may exacerbate those conditions.

In certain cases, decompression therapy may be recommended after back surgery if there are no hardware implants, such as metal screws or plates.

Epidural Steroid Injections (ESIs)

Epidural steroid injections are commonly used for leg and low back pain. Sometimes the injection alone will bring relief from pain. More commonly, however, the epidural steroid injection will be used in conjunction with a comprehensive treatment plan.

The main purpose of epidural steroid injections is to provide enough relief for the patient to begin exercise and stretching therapy.

Because steroid injections can have a negative effect on the organs, the doctor must be made aware if the patient has diabetes, congestive heart failure or kidney disease.

TENS for Sciatica

Transcutaneous Electrical Neural Stimulation, commonly referred to as TENS is regularly used to treat pain. Electrotherapy delivers small, but steady amounts of electricity to the affected areas.

This produces a sensation similar to pins and needles, but is not painful. TENS works because it interrupts the pain nerve signals so they do not reach the brain. When the affected area is free from pain, it causes the muscle to relax.

There are some conditions which, if present, TENS therapy should not be used. **In instances of pregnancy, cancer, if the patient has a pacemaker or poor sensation, TENS should not be used.** The downside of TENS treatments is that they may cause the patient to experience a false sense of well-being, which may result in over-exertion.

54

Chapter 5: Natural Remedies

Hypnosis

With hypnosis, the patient is placed in a mental state that allows the subconscious mind to receive suggestions easily. This is known as the Alpha state. The Alpha state occurs naturally just before sleep. During this state of mind, the patient experiences deep relaxation and is able to be taught how to respond to pain messages. Sometimes patients learn self-hypnosis for the purpose of pain reduction.

Always remember that pain is the body's way if signaling a person that something is wrong. If pain is present, there is usually a good reason for it. **Never attempt to eliminate the pain without finding out the cause.** Any type of therapy should be instituted only after medical diagnosis.

While in a hypnotic state, the patient is able to hear and receive suggestions regarding how to handle pain. Hypnosis works to address mental and physical causes of pain by training the body and mind appropriate responses to pain.

While under hypnosis, a patient can instruct the brain to release endorphins, which alleviate pain. This is similar to the feeling of euphoria that athletes experience during intense workouts. Hypnosis has actually been shown to expose emotional causes of pain, thereby providing ways in which healing can begin.

Hypnotherapy has also been known to improve sleep quality.

Yoga

The purpose of Yoga is to balance the spirit, mind and body. Some have received great relief from sciatica pain by using Yoga. The exercises are gentle and are designed to strengthen and stretch the muscles while creating body awareness. Yoga is an ancient practice for promoting relaxation through breathing and meditation exercises. Again, as some exercises may not be appropriate for every type of sciatica pain, a patient should always discuss this option with a physician prior to starting.

Reiki

Reiki is said to be a healing method involving spiritual energy. It is a very popular worldwide energy healing technique and is also referred to as 'hands on healing'. Reiki is based on the belief that all illness is related to excess or lack of energy in specific body organs or systems.

A practitioner of Reiki uses his or her hands through which life energy flows to treat the excess or deficiency of energy within a patient. The Reiki healing method is said to create a channel through which pure energy can flow. This energy is used to fill impaired systems or organs within the patient's aura.

Biofeedback

There is very little research on the effectiveness of biofeedback as relating to sciatica pain. It is a mind body therapy that teaches the patient to control or alter reactions to stress and pain. It uses visualization, mental images, physical movements and deep breathing

Massage Therapy

Since massage promotes the release of endorphins, it may be therapeutically beneficial to patients suffering from sciatica pain. Massage can also increase range of motion in the joints. Of course, massage should only be administered by a licensed healthcare professional with the consent of the patient's primary caregiver.

Naturopathy, Homeopathy, Herbal Medicine

There are many herbal and homeopathic treatments that claim to relieve pain and there are many books and other publications to help a person become knowledgeable and enable him or her to make an informed decision. There are also topical ointments, salves and gels that may provide relief, when directly applied to the affected area. If, however, the cause of pain is structural, these products may only bring short-term relief, at best.

Depending upon the root cause of the sciatica pain, in some cases, some natural remedies may help to alleviate pain. If, however, the root cause of pain is not diagnosed and resolved, any pain relief will only be temporary.

60

Chapter 6: Surgical Treatment Options

Back Surgery

Obviously, open back surgery is quite invasive, even to the point of requiring that some muscle tissue be peeled away from the spine. This is one of the reasons why recovery time for open back surgery is lengthy. In some cases, laser surgery is available and it may be a better option than open back surgery.

Usually, physicians and patients alike will agree that open back surgery only becomes an option if all else fails.

However, there are some conditions, in which surgery may be the most effective way to resolve the issue. Some of these conditions include the following

- Dysfunction of the bladder or bowel as a result of spinal cord compression

- Serious spinal stenosis that is not treatable non-surgically

- Neurologic conditions indicated by severe lower extremity weakness

- Symptoms that worsen

The three common types of surgery for sciatica pain are called discectomy, microdiscectomy, and laminectomy.

Any time the letters 'tomy' are at the end of a word, the word is referring to removal. A discectomy is exactly what it sounds like – removal of a herniated disk. In some cases only portions of the disk may need to be removed.

The difference between a discectomy and a microdiscectomy is that the microdiscectomy is minimally invasive surgery. A very small incision is made and through the use of microscopic magnification, the surgeon is able to insert very small instruments. A key benefit of minimally invasive surgery is that it greatly reduces the patient's recovery time.

Lamina is the name given to the thin bony shield that protects the spinal cord. The lamina is located on the inner arch of each vertebra. A laminectomy is when the lamina is removed from the vertebrae, thus, creating a space. This space reduces pressure and allows more room for the nerves to pass through the spine.

Surgery using robotics is become more sophisticated with time. It may be that the surgery needed can be done using minimally invasive techniques. Because of rapid advances in medicine, the assumption should never be made that minimally invasive surgery is not available. The patient should always discuss these possibilities with his or her physician.

Failed Back Surgery Syndrome

Unfortunately, some patients develop ongoing pain in the extremities or in the back following open back surgery. This is a possibility with any type of back surgery – whether laminectomy, discectomy or fusion.

Regardless of the cause, this condition is referred to by the medical community as Failed Back Surgery Syndrome or FBSS. The surgery, itself, may actually correct the condition for which it was intended. However, if it does not reduce the pain, it is considered FBSS.

There are complex measuring tools to determine the percent of patients who fall into the category of having FBSS. Likewise, in most cases, physicians may be able to determine the cause of FBSS, but may not have the knowledge or expertise to completely resolve the pain.

Sadly, sometimes a patient with FBSS may spend years trying to resolve continuing pain.

Chapter 7: Medications for Sciatica Pain

Depending upon the severity of sciatica pain, many patients find the need for some type of pain relief drug. It takes time to get an appointment with a primary care doctor, then more time to for tests, then additional time to see a specialist, if necessary.

If the patient suffers from severe sciatica pain, he or she may not be able to carry on the responsibilities of daily living. Severe sciatica pain can make even the most basic personal care tasks a nightmare. Even those who shun oral medication may find it necessary, at least until diagnosis had been made and treatment can begin.

Over-the-counter Pain Relief Medications

Pain relief medications fall into one of two categories. Some treat pain and inflammation, while others treat only pain. Both may work equally well in treating sciatica pain. In general, Non-Steroidal Anti-Inflammatory Drugs (NSAIDs) are the drug of choice in the treatment of sciatica pain. NSAIDs only control a limited amount of pain and may cause diarrhea, nausea and stomach ulcers.

NSAIDs should not be heavily relied upon for pain management and they should never be taken without eating.

Prescription Drugs

Extreme sciatica pain may only respond to prescription drugs. Your physician may prescribe an anti-inflammatory drug and a muscle relaxer. Narcotics may be recommended, for short-term pain relief, but they have dangerous side effects.

Other types of prescription medications used to treat severe sciatica pain are anticonvulsant drugs and anti-depressants. These two medications work by keeping pain signals from reaching the brain.

Natural Pain Relief for Sciatica

There are many and various forms of natural pain relief products. Ideally, the time to investigate the efficacy of these remedies would be prior to a sciatic episode. While these types of pain relievers may work, most people who are experiencing sciatica pain are not able to do the research necessary to implement a natural healing regimen. If, however, the patient is familiar with natural pain relief products, his or her physician may wholeheartedly endorse the use of these medications.

68

Chapter 8: Working with Sciatica Pain

Low back pain or worsening of back and neck problems can happen as a result of long periods of sitting an office chair. Prolonged sitting in the same position causes stress in the back, arms, shoulders, legs and neck.

When people tire from sitting, we naturally slouch, which causes the spinal ligaments to overstretch and places strain on disks and surrounding spinal tissues. If this is not corrected, this incorrect posture can result in damage to the spine and greater pain.

Creating Ideal Posture for the Office

An ergonomic office chair is a chair that can be adjusted to maximize back support and good sitting posture. These chairs allow each individual to adjust the chair, thus providing a custom fit.

Things to keep in mind when adjusting an office chair for correct ergonomics.

- Desk or workstation height must be considered when adjusting an office chair.

- Adjust the chair height so that the feet rest flat on the floor.

- While seated in the chair, adjust the lumbar support depth and height to your comfort.

- The chair recline allows each individual to adjust the back tension while moving back and forth. The chair back, however, should always provide consistent support, so should be slightly reclined, but not so reclined that it does not provide adequate support.

- The seat should be adjusted so that pressure is not applied to the back of the knees. There should be approximately an inch of seating on both sides of the legs.

- The armrest should be comfortable when the hands are at rest. Armrests should never be used while typing or using the mouse. Armrests should be lowered when not in use; otherwise, they may get in the way when typing.

Long Periods of Standing

If a person's job requires him or her to stand or walk all day, proper footwear is a must. Shoes should provide adequate space for the toes, proper arch and heel support.

Those who tend to have sore, achy feet may want to see a foot specialist to get professional advice about proper support or other issues you may have. Inadequate foot support often leads to back pain. Seeing a foot specialist may correct an issue that has the potential to cause pain or injury later.

72

Chapter 9: Travelling with Sciatica Pain

Sometimes people are hesitant about making vacation plans because their back pain can be so severe and unpredictable. Learn how to travel in order to take a much deserved vacation. Getting away to relax and enjoy yourself can actually be for the mind and body.

Actually, anxiety and stress of coping with sciatica pain may require getting away more often than those who do not have pain issues. Often, people with sciatica pain are discouraged from vacationing due to fear of a long trip or a strange bed. If you feel that you are unable to travel, your family will feel the impact because they will not want to take a vacation and leave you suffering at home.

There are actually ways to make your trip more enjoyable and even prevent sciatic episodes from happening. Listed below are some things you can do before and during a trip by air or car.

Before You Travel

- Ask your healthcare professional if you can travel with your condition.

- Look into the types of travel insurance that will address your specific needs.

- Make sure you carry enough medications to cover the duration of your stay and some additional days in the event there may be delays. It is very important to carry medications in the containers provided by the druggist with the original labels on them. Always keep medications with you in carry-on luggage. Everything you may need to care properly for your back should be packed in your carry-on luggage. Before booking your flight, it is a good idea to check with the airline about any new regulations regarding carry-on luggage.

- When traveling by air, book either first class or an aisle seat. This will give you easier access in getting into your seat and a little more room for stretching.

- Notify the airline in advance if you have special needs or need special accommodations.

- If travelling alone and may need assistance navigating the airport or getting to/from restrooms or even if you need help with your luggage, find out in advance if the airport can provide these services.

- The lighter you pace, the better. Preferably, use luggage on wheels and consider the option of purchasing toiletries when you get to your destination. If you are able to launder clothing, rather than pack for each day or your stay, you can avoid packing additional luggage.

- Learn about laundry facilities when selecting your accommodations.

- Take some music or meditation material to help you relax and reduce stress during the flight. This will help to ease tension and avoid stress and pain.

- Know your lodging's logistics. Find out if it will be easy to get around. Things to consider:

  1. Is there a medical facility available?
  2. How long is the trip from the airport to the lodging?
  3. Is it necessary to use any steps or stairways within the hotel?
  4. Does getting around require much walking?

Waiting for Transportation

- If you know that sitting seems to aggravate your condition, take advantage of the opportunity to walk, stand or stretch while waiting for your flight. Once your board the plane, opportunities to move around will be limited.

- In order to stay calm and relaxed, allow additional ground travel time. This will help you to avoid rushing and becoming stressed.

During a Flight

- People often overlook the need for ample hydration during a flight, particularly for someone taking back pain medication. Higher altitudes combined with some pain medications can cause the body to dehydrate more easily, which will contribute to back pain and disk issues. Try to avoid caffeine and alcohol, especially during the flight.

- At least hourly, try to stand and walk the aisles. You may even be able to do a few simple stretches.

- Wear loose-fitting, comfortable clothing

- If at all possible, try to stay awake during the flight. This will keep you moving and help you to avoid becoming stiff from sleeping in a cramped position.

- While seated, use a pillow for lumbar support. You can use a pillow or blanket to help support your back and make you as comfortable as possible.

- If you need assistance accessing overhead luggage compartments, ask for it.

Travelling by Car

Travelling by car can cause unbearable back, hip and leg pain to someone suffering from sciatica. This is due to limited mobility and sitting in a cramped space. Moving one foot/leg back and forth between the gas and brake pedal only serves to make matters even less comfortable.

Listed below are a few suggestions to make you more comfortable during road trips.

- Before your trip, try to determine at what intervals you need to stop for breaks. Get to know how long you can drive comfortably before you need to get out of the car and move around.

- Take advantage of restroom breaks and gas station stops to move around and stretch for at least ten minutes.

- Sitting on a mobile phone or wallet in the back pocket can cause an abnormal position that lifts one hip higher. Remember to remove bulky items from pack pockets.

- Vehicle built-in supports should be adjusted to meet your individual needs. If a lumbar support seat is not available, place a pillow in the lumbar region of your back for support.

- Make use of the vehicle's heated seats, if available. If the vehicle does not have heated seats, you may be able to purchase a heating pad that will be appropriate for travel.

- Remember to hydrate by drinking water during the trip and try to eat healthy snacks.

- Drink plenty of water during the journey; it is easy to get dehydrated which is not good for you or your back. Try to eat healthy nutritious snacks.

- When you arrive at your destination, take a warm bath or shower. This will help relax tense muscles.

Chapter 10: Sleeping with Sciatica Pain

The Right Mattress

Of course, a good night's sleep is essential to our well-being. Sciatica pain may worsen if you are sleeping on the wrong mattress. We all want to be comfy and cozy, but a mattress that gives proper support helps maintain good sleeping posture, lessens muscle strain and keeps the spine in proper alignment. However, comfort should not be compromised by selecting a mattress that is too firm.

Listed below are some basic guidelines for selecting a mattress that provides both comfort and support.

Rule Number 1:

There is no such thing as "the best mattress on the market" for you. Yes, there are various quality mattresses, but buying a mattress that is top of the line will not guarantee a good night's sleep. Always, always look for a mattress that meets your individual needs for comfort and support.

Rule Number 2:

Do some research and understand how a mattress is constructed. Some mattresses use inner springs or coils to provide support. The number of coils used varies from mattress to mattress. In addition, padding which covers the inner springs can range anywhere from 7 to 8 inch thick. These factors should be considered when selecting a mattress.

Rule Number 3:

Look for a mattress with back support and comfort. Natural alignment and curve of the spine should always be supported by a good mattress. The correct level of back support will keep the patient from having muscle pain in the morning. Do not rule out a mattress that is labeled 'medium' support. This may be exactly what you need, but you won't know if you don't try it.

Rule Number 4:

Know when your mattress is worn out: If your bed is lumpy or sags in the middle, or if you can feel the inner coils, most likely it is time to get a new mattress. Using a board to support a sagging mattress may be a short-term fix just until a new mattress can be purchased

The Right Position

How should a sciatica pain sufferer sleep? Achieving comfort is our goal in getting a good night's rest.

Here are some things you might want to consider:

- Many with back pain and sciatica find that sleeping on the side and placing a pillow between the knees helps to reduce pressure on the lower back.

- For those suffering from bilateral sciatica pain, another pointer is to sleep on the side that is pain free.

- Some might want to use a full body pillow. Some people find them very useful in maintaining head, neck and spine alignment during sleep.

- For those who prefer to sleep on their backs, try placing a small pillow or towel at the waist. This will help with lumbar support. Back sleepers also use a pillow under the knees.

- Some physicians advise against sleeping on the stomach because it can cause pressure and tension in the back.

- For patients recovering from surgery, it is best to consult the surgeon for advice on how to sleep.

Chapter 11: Myths and Facts about Sciatica

As is the case with everything, certainly, all facts and myths have gray areas if we look hard enough. The following statements are general consensus, rather than cold hard facts.

Myth: Finding the cure for sciatica is difficult.
Fact: Accurate diagnosis is difficult – not finding a cure.

Myth: Sciatica is harmful.
Fact: Sciatica is a symptom of potentially harmful conditions.

Myth: Back injuries never completely heal.
Fact: Correct diagnosis and treatment can lead to total healing depending upon the cause.

Myth: Lifting causes sciatica.

Fact: Lifting done incorrectly may cause sciatica or other back issues.

Myth: Complete bed rest helps sciatica pain.
Fact: Short-term bed rest is helpful, but long-term bed rest can prove more harmful than good.

Myth: With sciatica, it is better to stand than sit.
Fact: Prolonged sitting and standing both weigh on the lumbar spine; however, many sciatica patients report that sitting is more painful than standing.

Summary: Learn to Say Sayonara Sciatica

We have covered much useful material, thus far. In this chapter, we will highlight several key things to remember about becoming free from sciatica pain. Often times, it is a slow process, but following simple instructions can help resolve pain issues and rejuvenate active lifestyles.

1) Seek medical attention

If a week has gone by since the onset of your sciatica pain and you have tried several home remedies and the pain is the same or worse, it is time to see your doctor. Whenever there is undiagnosed pain, there is the possibility of causing further injury. In addition, the more time lapse between onset and treatment, the longer the recovery period.

2) Learn about your condition

Sometimes a person will visit the doctor, return home, and not be able to answer any questions about what the doctor said. We all have a responsibility to ourselves to be attentive to what the doctor is saying. Do know allow any healthcare professional to cause you to feel rushed. It is imperative that every patient understands his or her condition. In most cases, the physician is more than willing to consult with you. If you do not understand an explanation, ask for further clarification. Remember, there is no such thing as a stupid question.

3) Embrace your uniqueness

My father had a bad habit of asking several people about the same concern. Maybe some had experienced his concern – and some had not. At the end of the day, he would have several different opinions from people who had experienced his concern in several different ways. He would be frustrated and so would I.

Each of us is a designer's original. We are similar, yet different. We have unique fingerprints and vocal patterns and retina scans and only God knows what else. We are all the same, but different. Each patient should expect his or her personal experience with sciatica pain and treatment to be just that – unique and personal.

4) Listen to your body, but don't over-pamper

For the most part, people avoid any kind of exertion at the onset of sciatica pain. If you rest too long, the body will let you know that you need to move around. The muscles will become stiff from lack of use, at which point it is telling you that it is time to get up and move... and yes, it may hurt a little, but it is absolutely necessary to bring about healing. Conversely, do not over-exercise. Strive for a balance and perhaps, a gradual increase in pace and intensity. The most effective exercises for sciatica pain are done slowly and methodically. Gentle stretching is very important

5) Follow advice of healthcare professionals

I can't tell you how many times I've heard people complain about their back pain. When asked if they were given exercises, most respond, "Oh, yes." When asked if they actually do the exercises prescribed, the answer is usually, "Oh, I don't have time for that." If the patient isn't going to do what is prescribed, he or she shouldn't complain about on-going pain. Yes, sometimes exercise may be uncomfortable. By nature, stretching and realignment will cause discomfort, because the muscle and other tissues have become tight. Exercise, when done as prescribed, can be very beneficial in relieving sciatica pain.

Anything and everything must be maintained. If the doctor prescribed exercise treatment for sciatica pain, it needs to be done. Patients need to do their part to attain better conditioning for their backs. This means "Do your exercises."

6) Talk to your healthcare professionals about alternative treatment

What should you do if your doctor does not recommend a treatment you feel may be beneficial to your condition? Conversely, what if he recommends a treatment with which you are not comfortable? I cannot stress enough the importance of open, clear communication with your healthcare professional. Consultation is a big part of being a physician. It is up to you, however, to ensure that you fully understand the diagnosis, the proposed treatment options and prognosis. You may need to ask a friend or relative to attend a consultation so that you and your physician are in complete agreement.

7) Institute lifestyle changes – posture, lumbar support options, etc.

Let's say that you have recently been afflicted with gradually increasing sciatica pain on your left side. It just so happens that, for as long as you can remember, you have crossed your right leg when sitting. There is a strong possibility that you may need to stop crossing your right leg, yes? Lifestyle changes are never easy, but when we make a conscious effort, we can make changes that will have a positive impact on our lives.

8) Be positive and patient

Whether the sciatica pain came as a direct result from injury or if it came on more gradually, attitude can play a major role in outcome. Most of us have heard the saying, "If you think you can't, you can't." It is a true statement. My sciatica pain was not resolved until I decided that I would not allow it to ruin and dominate my life. My first step in healing was to stop focusing all thought and energy on the pain and begin to examine the source of the pain and how to resolve the root cause. Negative thinking affects all aspects of our lives, and healing is no different.

Once you have decided that sciatica pain will NOT take over your life, apply the treatments that are appropriate for you and begin to look for signs of improvement. No matter how small, rejoice in every positive turn. If you were able to walk just two minutes longer today than yesterday, rejoice. If you were able to take a ride in your car with diminished pain, acknowledge that accomplishment and rejoice. If it turns out that current treatment is not helping, look forward to trying alternative treatment. No, the pain will not go away overnight, but believe that it WILL go away.

I have been a liturgical dance leader for several years, and there have been times when I thought, "I'm not going to be able to dance." In spite of that nagging doubt, I continued to see myself dancing, and guess what? I am STILL dancing because I exercised my faith and I believed that the pain WOULD go away.

9) Stretch regularly

Picture a brand new balloon. What is the first thing we do before trying to blow it up? Yes, we stretch it. When we stretch a balloon, we are applying tension, but each time we release the tension, the balloon become less tight and able to expand without popping. This is what stretching does for our muscles and tendons. Stretching the hamstrings does absolute wonders for low back pain because it loosens tension on the back muscles.

10) Avoid activities known to cause recurring issues

If you have been diagnosed with a herniated disk or other structural condition of the spine, you will probably need to avoid activities that will worsen this condition. Through learning about the condition and consulting with your healthcare professional, you will be able to determine what activities you may need to avoid.

11) Grow old gracefully

In our youth-oriented society, we sometimes forget that it's OK to grow older. There are fringe benefits and blessings at every age, although sometimes we need a closer look to see them. Older bones and muscles may not be as strong as they used to be. We may find the need to modify some activities to accommodate these physical changes. Facing these changes can enable us to live active lives longer. Conversely, if we ignore these changes and do not use appropriate care and caution, we may actually contribute to the possibility of debilitating damage and injury.

Printed in Great Britain
by Amazon

50749915R00058